MW00882881

KIDNEY DISEASE
FOOD LIST AND FOOD GUIDE
2024

Comprehensive guide on what to eat and limit with Low Potassium, Low Phosphorus, and Low Sodium Recipes for Kidney patient

Dr. JANE THORNTHWAITE

TABLE OF CONTENTS

3

Chapter 1

Understanding Kidney Disease

The Role of Kidneys in Your Health

The kidneys are vital organs that act as the body's natural filtration system, playing a critical role in maintaining overall health. They work tirelessly to remove waste products and toxins from the bloodstream, which are then excreted through urine. Beyond waste elimination, kidneys are instrumental in managing the body's fluid balance, ensuring that water and electrolyte levels remain in harmony to support cell function. They also regulate blood pressure by controlling fluid volume and releasing hormones that adjust blood vessel constriction. Additionally, kidneys maintain the body's acid-base balance, ensuring metabolic processes proceed smoothly. They produce erythropoietin, a hormone essential for the production of red blood cells, supporting oxygen transport throughout the body. Moreover, kidneys help keep bones healthy by converting vitamin D into its active form, aiding calcium absorption. Their role extends to metabolic functions, such as breaking down medications and helping regulate blood sugar levels during fasting. Given their wide-ranging responsibilities, maintaining kidney health is paramount, as their dysfunction can lead to significant health issues, emphasizing the importance of a healthy diet, adequate hydration, and regular check-ups to ensure these vital organs function optimally.

Introduction to Kidney Disease

Kidney disease refers to a condition where the kidneys are damaged and cannot perform their essential functions effectively. This damage can accumulate over time, leading to a decrease in the kidney's ability to filter out waste and excess fluids from the body. As a result, harmful substances can build up in the blood, leading to various health issues. Kidney disease can stem from multiple causes, including high blood pressure, diabetes, and other chronic conditions that put a strain on the kidneys. In its early stages, kidney disease often goes unnoticed because it can be asymptomatic or present with non-specific symptoms. However, as the disease progresses, it can lead to more serious complications like hypertension, anemia, weak bones, poor nutritional health, and nerve damage. The advanced stage of kidney disease, known as kidney failure or end-stage renal disease, requires significant medical intervention, such as dialysis or a kidney transplant, to perform the functions of the kidneys. Early detection and management through lifestyle changes and medication can help slow the progression of kidney disease and maintain overall health.

Causes and Types of Kidney Disease

Kidney disease can arise from various causes, affecting the kidneys' ability to function properly. It is generally classified into two main types: acute kidney injury (AKI) and chronic kidney disease (CKD), each with distinct causes and progression patterns.

Acute kidney injury is a sudden loss of kidney function that occurs within a few hours or days, often as a result of reduced blood flow to the kidneys, direct damage to the kidneys themselves, or blockage of the urinary tract that prevents urine from leaving the body. Causes of AKI include severe or sudden dehydration, toxic kidney injury from poisons or certain medications, and acute blockage of the urinary tract.

Chronic kidney disease, on the other hand, develops over many years and is mainly caused by long-term conditions that put a strain on the kidneys. The leading causes of CKD include diabetes, which damages the nephrons in the kidneys through high blood sugar levels, and high blood pressure, which puts extra pressure on the small blood vessels in the kidneys, damaging them over time. Other causes include autoimmune diseases, genetic disorders like polycystic kidney disease, prolonged urinary tract obstruction, and recurrent kidney infections. Both types of kidney disease can lead to a buildup of waste products in the body, causing various health problems. Early detection and treatment can help manage the symptoms of kidney disease and slow its progression, emphasizing the importance of regular check-ups for those at risk

How Your Diet Affects Kidney Disease

Your diet plays a significant role in managing and affecting the progression of kidney disease. The kidneys are responsible for filtering waste products and excess fluids from the blood, and what you eat and drink directly impacts your workload and efficiency. A diet that is high in certain nutrients can strain the kidneys, accelerating the progression of kidney disease, while a carefully planned diet can help manage the disease's symptoms and slow its progression.

High levels of sodium, potassium, and phosphorus in the diet can be particularly challenging for individuals with kidney disease. The kidneys regulate these minerals in the body, but when they're not functioning properly, these minerals can build up to unhealthy levels. A high sodium intake can increase blood pressure, worsening kidney damage. Potassium and phosphorus need to be carefully managed as well, as imbalances can lead to heart problems and bone disease, respectively.

Protein intake is another critical dietary consideration. While protein is an essential nutrient, kidneys in a diseased state may struggle to eliminate the waste products of protein metabolism. This doesn't mean protein should be avoided entirely, but rather consumed in moderation, with guidance from healthcare professionals to determine the right amount.

Moreover, a diet high in processed and fast foods can contribute to health issues like hypertension and type 2 diabetes, both of which are risk factors for developing kidney disease. On the other hand, a diet rich in fruits, vegetables, whole grains, and lean proteins can support kidney health by providing essential nutrients without overburdening the kidneys.

Fluid intake must also be monitored, especially in the later stages of kidney disease, as the kidneys' ability to balance the body's fluids is compromised. Too much fluid can lead to swelling, high blood pressure, and heart problems, while too little can cause dehydration.

Adopting a kidney-friendly diet can help control the accumulation of waste products and fluids, reduce kidney disease symptoms, and potentially slow the progression of the disease. It often involves limiting certain nutrients while ensuring the diet is nutritionally balanced, and tailored to the individual's stage of kidney disease, overall health, and lifestyle. Consulting with a dietitian who specializes in kidney disease is crucial to creating a diet plan that meets these needs.

Chapter 2

Special Considerations in Your Diet

Managing Protein Intake

Managing protein intake is crucial for individuals with kidney disease, as the kidneys are responsible for filtering the by-products of protein metabolism. While protein is essential for health, consuming it in excessive amounts can overburden diseased kidneys, leading to further damage. The key is to consume high-quality protein in moderation. High-quality proteins, such as egg whites, poultry, fish, and plant-based options like quinoa and soy products, provide essential amino acids with less phosphorus, making them better choices for kidney health. The amount of protein needed varies depending on the stage of kidney disease, body size, and overall health. It's important to work with a healthcare provider or dietitian to determine the right amount of protein for your individual needs. This personalized approach helps ensure that the body gets the nutrients it needs without putting extra strain on the kidneys, aiding in the management of kidney disease and preserving kidney function.

The Role of Potassium and Phosphorus

Potassium and phosphorus are essential minerals that play critical roles in the body but require careful management in individuals with kidney disease. Potassium is vital for nerve function, muscle control, and heart health. However, when the kidneys cannot efficiently remove excess potassium, it can accumulate in the blood, potentially leading to dangerous heart rhythms. Phosphorus, on the other hand, is important for building and repairing bones and teeth, maintaining proper muscle function, and supporting cell health. But, like potassium, when kidney function declines, phosphorus can build up in the body, leading to bone and cardiovascular issues. Managing intake of these minerals through diet becomes crucial for those with kidney disease to prevent hyperkalemia (high potassium levels) and hyperphosphatemia (high phosphorus levels), which can exacerbate health problems. Healthcare providers often recommend diets low in these minerals and may prescribe medication to help control their levels in the blood, maintaining balance and protecting overall health

Recommended Fluid Intake:

For individuals with kidney disease, managing fluid intake is crucial to prevent complications such as fluid overload, which can strain the heart and lungs, and contribute to hypertension and swelling. The recommended fluid intake can vary significantly depending on the stage of kidney disease, treatment methods such as dialysis, and individual factors including remaining kidney function, daily urine output, and the presence of conditions like heart failure. Typically, those with advanced kidney disease or on dialysis may need to restrict their fluid intake more strictly to avoid the risks associated with fluid retention. It's important to include not just water but also other beverages and foods with high water content in the total daily fluid intake. Consulting with a healthcare professional or a dietitian is essential to determine an appropriate fluid intake that balances hydration needs without overburdening the kidneys, taking into account personal health status and lifestyle.

Vitamins and Minerals in Kidney Disease

In kidney disease, the balance of vitamins and minerals can be significantly disrupted, necessitating careful management to avoid deficiencies and toxicities. Since the kidneys play a crucial role in filtering and balancing minerals and vitamins, their dysfunction can lead to imbalances. For instance, vitamin B and D levels often become deficient in kidney disease patients due to decreased absorption and the kidneys' inability to convert vitamin D to its active form. Conversely, minerals like potassium and phosphorus can accumulate to harmful levels since the kidneys cannot excrete them efficiently.

Patients may need to adjust their diet or take supplements specifically designed for people with kidney disease, avoiding standard multivitamins due to high levels of certain minerals like potassium and phosphorus. It's important to consult healthcare providers before starting any supplements, as some can further harm kidney function. Tailored nutritional management, including careful monitoring of vitamin and mineral intake, is essential for managing kidney disease and maintaining overall health.

Chapter 3

Kidney-Friendly food list

Foods to Eat: A Comprehensive List

Managing kidney disease involves a careful selection of foods to support kidney health while minimizing the kidneys' workload. A kidney-friendly diet typically focuses on low-sodium, low-potassium, and low-phosphorus choices, along with the appropriate amount of high-quality protein. Here's a guide on foods to eat for those managing kidney disease, aimed at providing variety and nutrition without overburdening the kidneys.

Fruits

- **Apples**: High in fiber and anti-inflammatory properties, apples are a good choice for a kidney diet.

25

- **Berries**: Blueberries, strawberries, and raspberries are rich in antioxidants and vitamins, with relatively low potassium levels.
- **Cherries**: Known for their anti-inflammatory properties, cherries are a kidney-friendly snack.
- **Grapes**: Grapes are high in antioxidants and vitamin C, making them a healthy choice for kidney health.

Vegetables

- **Cauliflower**: This versatile vegetable is high in vitamin C and contains compounds that can help neutralize toxic substances in the body.
- **Garlic**: Adds flavor to dishes without the need for salt, and has natural anti-inflammatory properties.

- **Onions**: Another excellent flavor enhancer, onions are low in potassium and high in antioxidants.
- **Red bell peppers**: Low in potassium and high in vitamins C, A, and B6, red bell peppers are great for kidney health.
- **Cabbage**: A cruciferous vegetable that's low in potassium and rich in vitamins K and C, and fiber.

Proteins

- **Egg whites**: High-quality protein source that's lower in phosphorus than other protein sources like egg yolks.
- **Fish**: Certain fish like salmon, mackerel, and herring are good sources of omega-3 fatty acids but should be consumed in moderation due to their potassium content.

- **Chicken**: A lean protein choice that's lower in fat and phosphorus than red meats, making it a better option for kidney health.

Grains

- **White rice, pasta, and bread**: These have lower fiber than their whole-grain counterparts but are generally lower in phosphorus and potassium.
- **Buckwheat and bulgur**: These grains are good alternatives to other higher phosphorus grains.

Dairy and Dairy Alternatives

- **Rice milk or almond milk**: Lower in phosphorus and potassium than cow's milk, these alternatives can be suitable for a kidney diet.
- **Non-dairy creamers and unenriched rice milk**: Can be used in place of traditional dairy products.

Beverages

- **Water**: The best choice for staying hydrated while keeping kidney health in check.

- **Clear sodas and lemon-lime beverages**: Generally lower in potassium and phosphorus than other sodas.

Other Considerations

- **Herbs and spices**: Use these to flavor foods instead of salt.

- **Small portions of lower-potassium fruits and vegetables**: Moderation is key, even with kidney-friendly foods.

Foods to Avoid or Limit

When managing kidney disease, certain foods can exacerbate the condition by increasing the workload on the kidneys or contributing to fluid and waste buildup in the body Here's a list of foods to avoid or limit if you have kidney disease:

High-Sodium Foods

- **Processed and Packaged Foods**: Many canned soups, frozen dinners, and snack foods are high in sodium, which can increase blood pressure and worsen kidney function.

- **Deli Meats and Cured Meats**: These are often loaded with sodium for preservation.

- **Salted Snacks**: Chips, pretzels, and crackers typically have high sodium content.

High-Potassium Foods

- **Certain Fruits and Vegetables**: Avocados, bananas, oranges, potatoes, tomatoes, and spinach are high in potassium, which can be harmful in excess if your kidneys are not functioning properly.

- **Whole Grains**: Brown rice, whole wheat bread, and bran cereals contain more potassium than their refined counterparts.

High-Phosphorus Foods

- **Dairy Products**: Milk, cheese, yogurt, and ice cream are high in phosphorus and should be limited.

- **Nuts and Seeds**: Including almonds, peanuts, sunflower seeds, and pumpkin seeds.

- **Beans and Lentils**: These are nutritious but high in phosphorus, so intake should be moderated.

Protein-Rich Foods

While not all protein-rich foods need to be avoided, those with kidney disease may need to limit their overall protein intake, especially from sources high in phosphorus and sodium.

- **Red Meat**: Beef, pork, and lamb are not only high in protein but also phosphorus and saturated fats.

- **Certain Seafoods**: Some types of fish and shellfish are high in phosphorus.

Others

- **Dark Colas**: These sodas contain high levels of phosphorus due to the phosphoric acid used for flavoring.

- **Chocolate**: High in phosphorus and potassium.

- **Processed Grains**: Such as those found in ready-to-eat cereals, may also be fortified with minerals.

- **Alcohol**: This can affect electrolyte balance and overall fluid volume in your body.

Beverages

- **Beverages with Added Minerals**: Some bottled or flavored waters may have added electrolytes or minerals that can affect kidney health

Chapter 4

Planning Your Kidney Disease Diet

Setting Up Your Kitchen for Success

Setting up your kitchen for success, especially when managing kidney disease, involves creating an environment that supports a kidney-friendly diet. This preparation can make dietary changes easier to implement and maintain.

Here are some strategies to consider:

1.   **Stock Up on Kidney-Friendly Foods**: Fill your pantry and refrigerator with foods low in sodium, potassium, and phosphorus. Prioritize fresh fruits and vegetables, lean proteins like poultry and fish, whole grains, and low-phosphorus dairy alternatives.

2.   **Organize for Easy Access**: Arrange your kitchen so that kidney-friendly options

are the most accessible. This setup encourages making healthier choices.

3.	**Herbs and Spices Over Salt**: Replace salt with a variety of herbs and spices to flavor your meals without increasing sodium intake. Consider growing a small herb garden in your kitchen for fresh herbs.

4.	**Limit Unhealthy Temptations**: Keep foods high in sodium, potassium, and phosphorus—such as processed snacks, canned goods with added salt, and dairy products—out of sight or off your shopping list to avoid temptation.

5.	**Cookware and Tools**: Invest in non-stick cookware to reduce the need for cooking oils and salt. Having a good set of knives, cutting boards, and storage containers can make meal prep easier and more appealing.

6.   **Label Reading Area**: Create a space where you can comfortably read food labels while sorting your groceries. This practice can help you become more familiar with the nutritional content of foods and make better choices.

7.   **Meal Prep Stations**: Designate areas for washing, chopping, and preparing foods. Keeping these tasks organized can streamline meal preparation and make it less of a chore.

8.   **Healthy Recipe Resources**: Keep a collection of kidney-friendly recipes readily available, whether in a binder, a cookbook, or saved online, to inspire and guide your meal planning.

9.   **Stay Hydrated**: Set up a hydration station with a water filter pitcher or bottles of water to remind you to drink fluids

regularly, within the limits recommended for your condition.

Meal Planning Strategies

Meal planning is a vital strategy for managing kidney disease, helping to ensure that dietary restrictions are met while still enjoying a variety of nutritious and tasty meals. Effective meal planning can alleviate the stress of daily decisions about what to eat, control nutrient intake, and maintain overall health.

Here are key strategies for successful meal planning:

1. **Understand Dietary Needs**: Familiarize yourself with the specific dietary requirements for kidney disease, including limits on sodium, potassium, phosphorus, and protein. Knowing which foods to focus

on and which to limit is the foundation of meal planning.

2.   **Consult with a Dietitian**: A dietitian specializing in kidney disease can provide personalized advice on dietary needs and help create a meal plan that fits your lifestyle, taste preferences, and nutritional requirements.

3.   **Plan Your Meals Weekly**: Allocate time each week to plan your meals, including main dishes and sides. Planning can help you ensure variety and balance in your diet.

4.   **Create a Shopping List**: Based on your meal plan, make a shopping list to avoid impulse buys and ensure you have all the necessary ingredients for your kidney-friendly meals.

5.   **Prep in Advance**: Prepare ingredients or entire meals in advance to save time and

reduce the temptation to opt for less healthy options. Cooking in batches and storing portions for later can also help manage portion sizes and make meal times simpler.

6.   **Portion Control**: Be mindful of portion sizes, especially for foods high in potassium, phosphorus, and sodium. Use measuring cups and scales to ensure accurate portions that align with your dietary needs.

7.   **Incorporate Variety**: To prevent dietary boredom, include a variety of foods within your dietary restrictions. Experiment with different herbs and spices to add flavor without adding sodium.

8.   **Mind Fluid Intake**: If your fluid intake needs to be monitored, plan not just for solid meals but also account for soups, beverages, and foods high in water content.

9.   **Read Labels**: When shopping, always read food labels to check for hidden sources of sodium, potassium, and phosphorus. This habit is crucial for sticking to your dietary guidelines.

10.   **Flexible Meals**: Plan meals that can be easily adjusted to fit the needs of others in your household without having to prepare separate dishes.

Preparing Kidney-Friendly Meals at Home

Preparing kidney-friendly meals at home involves the mindful selection of ingredients and cooking methods to create dishes that support kidney health while being flavorful and satisfying. Here are essential tips for cooking kidney-friendly meals that cater to the dietary needs of those with kidney disease:

Choose Low-Sodium Alternatives

- **Herbs and Spices**: Use fresh or dried herbs, spices, and sodium-free seasoning blends instead of salt to add flavor to your dishes.

- **Homemade Stocks and Broths**: Make your stocks and broths to control the sodium content, avoiding store-bought versions that are often high in sodium.

Opt for Low-Potassium Vegetables and Fruits

- **Vegetable Choices**: Focus on vegetables like cauliflower, bell peppers, cabbage, and apples, which are lower in potassium compared to others like potatoes, tomatoes, and bananas.

- **Leaching**: For vegetables that are higher in potassium, consider

41

leaching them to remove some of the potassium. This involves cutting the vegetables into small pieces, soaking them in water for several hours, and then cooking them in fresh water.

Control Phosphorus Intake

- **Dairy Alternatives**: Use rice milk, almond milk, or other non-dairy alternatives that are low in phosphorus, compared to regular dairy products.

- **Limit Processed Foods**: Many processed foods contain added phosphates as preservatives. Opt for fresh or homemade options when possible.

Include High-Quality Protein

- **Lean Proteins**: Incorporate sources of high-quality protein such as chicken, fish, and egg whites, which are easier on the kidneys than red meats.

- **Portion Control**: Be mindful of portion sizes to avoid consuming too much protein.

Cooking Methods

- **Grilling, Baking, and Steaming**: These cooking methods do not require added fat and can enhance the natural flavors of foods without the need for excessive seasoning.

- **Sautéing**: Use a non-stick pan and a small amount of olive oil or cooking spray to reduce the need for added fats and salt.

Focus on Whole Foods

- **Whole Grains**: Choose whole grains like buckwheat, bulgur, and rice, which are generally lower in phosphorus than processed grains.

- **Fresh Ingredients**: Build meals around fresh ingredients to avoid the hidden sodium, potassium, and phosphorus in processed foods.

Hydration

- **Fluid Management**: If you need to manage fluid intake, be mindful of the water content in soups, stews, and fruits, and adjust your fluid intake accordingly.

Meal Planning

- **Plan Ahead**: Planning meals can help ensure that you have the appropriate ingredients on hand, reducing the temptation to opt for less kidney-friendly options.
- **Diverse Recipes**: Explore a variety of kidney-friendly recipes to keep meals interesting and ensure a balance of nutrients.

Eating Out with Kidney Disease

Eating out with kidney disease can be challenging due to less control over ingredients and cooking methods, which can affect dietary restrictions. However, with careful planning and informed choices, dining out can still be an enjoyable experience without compromising kidney health. Here are strategies to navigate eating out:

Plan Ahead

- **Research the Restaurant**: Look up the menu online beforehand to find kidney-friendly options. Some restaurants may offer nutritional information, making it easier to choose dishes that fit within your dietary restrictions.

- **Call Ahead**: Don't hesitate to call the restaurant and ask about their ability to accommodate special dietary needs. Many are willing to modify dishes to meet your requirements.

Make Informed Menu Choices

- **Sodium**: Opt for dishes that are likely to be lower in sodium, such as grilled or roasted meats and vegetables, and over-processed or fried foods. Request no added salt.

- **Potassium and Phosphorus**: Avoid high-potassium foods like potatoes, tomatoes, and avocados, and high-phosphorus foods like dairy and nuts. Salads with leafy greens and low-potassium vegetables are often a safe bet but watch out for dressings and add-ons.

- **Protein**: Choose lean protein sources and be mindful of portion sizes. Fish and poultry are often better choices than red meats.

Request Modifications

- **Sauce and Dressing on the Side**: This gives you control over the amount you consume, reducing your intake of hidden sodium, potassium, and phosphorus.

- **Modify Side Dishes**: Ask for substitutions for high-potassium side dishes, like swapping out French fries for a salad or steamed vegetables.

Portion Control

- **Share Meals**: Restaurant portions can be large. Consider sharing a dish with a dining companion to manage portion sizes and nutrient intake.

- **Box It Up**: Another strategy is to ask for a to-go box right away and set aside half of your meal for later.

Stay Hydrated

- **Beverage Choices**: Stick with water or other low-potassium beverages. Avoid or limit high-phosphate drinks like cola and opt for clear sodas or lemonade if you desire something other than water.

Communicate with Your Server

- **Be Specific**: Communicate your dietary needs to your server. Most restaurants are accustomed to handling special requests and can guide you to the safest choices on the menu.

Enjoy Your Meal Mindfully

- **Savor Your Food**: Eating out is an experience. Enjoy the flavors and the company you're with, eating slowly and mindfully to make the most of your dining out experience.

Chapter 5

28-day Meal plan for Kidney disease Patient

This 28-day meal plan is a guide and should be adjusted based on individual dietary needs, preferences, and any specific medical advice from healthcare providers.

Week 1

Day 1

- Breakfast: Low-Sodium Oatmeal with Apples and Cinnamon

- Lunch: Quinoa Salad with Chickpeas and Cucumbers

- Dinner: Lemon Herb Baked Cod with Steamed Broccoli

- Snack: Cucumber and Hummus Bites

- Dessert: Berry and Yogurt Parfait

Day 2

- Breakfast: Egg White Scramble with Spinach and Bell Peppers

- Lunch: Grilled Chicken Breast with Steamed Broccoli

- Dinner: Garlic Olive Oil Pasta with Spinach

- Snack: Apple Slices with Almond Butter

- Dessert: Apple Cinnamon Baked Apples

Day 3

- Breakfast: Blueberry Almond Breakfast Quinoa

- Lunch: Vegetable Stir-Fry with Tofu

- Dinner: Turkey and Quinoa Stuffed Peppers

- Snack: Carrot Sticks with Avocado Dip

- Dessert: Angel Food Cake with Fresh Berries

Day 4

- Breakfast: Avocado Toast on Whole Grain Bread

- Lunch: Tuna Salad Sandwich on Whole Wheat Bread

- Dinner: Baked Chicken with Roasted Carrots and Parsnips

- Snack: Baked Kale Chips

- Dessert: Peach Sorbet

Day 5

- Breakfast: Banana Yogurt Smoothie

- Lunch: Roasted Turkey and Avocado Wrap

- Dinner: Salmon Salad with Mixed Greens

- Snack: Zucchini Muffins

- Dessert: Rice Pudding

Day 6

- Breakfast: Cottage Cheese with Pineapple

- Lunch: Lentil Soup

- Dinner: Chicken and Broccoli Stir-Fry

- Snack: Rice Cakes with Cottage Cheese and Cherry Tomatoes

- Dessert: Vanilla and Almond Mousse

Day 7

- Breakfast: Zucchini Bread Muffins

- Lunch: Grilled Veggie and Hummus Sandwich

- Dinner: Beef and Mushroom Skillet

- Snack: Roasted Chickpeas

- Dessert: Carrot Cake Muffins

Week 2

Day 8

- Breakfast: Cottage Cheese with Pineapple

- Lunch: Peach and Cottage Cheese Pancakes

- Dinner: Chicken and Avocado Salad

- Snack: Greek Yogurt with Berries

- Dessert: Chocolate Avocado Pudding

Day 9

- Breakfast: Almond Butter and Banana Sandwich

- Lunch: Spinach and Goat Cheese Salad

- Dinner: Baked Salmon with Asparagus

- Snack: Boiled Eggs

- Dessert: Baked Pears with Honey and Walnuts

Day 10

- Breakfast: Spinach and Mushroom Omelette

- Lunch: Cauliflower Rice Stir-Fry

- Dinner: Eggplant Parmesan (Light Version)

- Snack: Peanut Butter Banana Roll-Ups

- Dessert: Strawberry Banana Smoothie

Day 11

- Breakfast: Apple Cinnamon Baked Oatmeal

- Lunch: Beet and Goat Cheese Arugula Salad

- Dinner: Shrimp and Asparagus Risotto

- Snack: Avocado Toast with Egg

- Dessert: Lemon Ricotta Blueberry Cupcakes

Day 12

- Breakfast: Repeat your favorite breakfast from the previous days

- Lunch: Turkey and Avocado Wrap

- Dinner: Vegetable Lentil Stew

- Snack: Veggie Sticks with Greek Yogurt Ranch Dip

- Dessert: Almond Joy Bars (Kidney-Friendly Version)

Day 13

- Breakfast: Blueberry Almond Breakfast Quinoa

- Lunch: Grilled Veggie and Hummus Sandwich

- Dinner: Baked Lemon Pepper Tilapia

- Snack: Cucumber and Hummus Bites

- Dessert: Angel Food Cake with Fresh Berries

Day 14

- Breakfast: Egg White Scramble with Spinach and Bell Peppers

- Lunch: Quinoa Salad with Chickpeas and Cucumbers

- Dinner: Garlic Olive Oil Pasta with Spinach

- Snack: Apple Slices with Almond Butter

- Dessert: Berry and Yogurt Parfait

Week 3

Day 15

- Breakfast: Avocado Toast on Whole Grain Bread

- Lunch: Lentil Soup

- Dinner: Grilled Vegetable Platter

- Snack: Greek Yogurt with Berries

- Dessert: Apple Cinnamon Baked Apples

Day 16

- Breakfast: Banana Yogurt Smoothie

- Lunch: Spinach and Goat Cheese Salad

- Dinner: Turkey and Quinoa Stuffed Peppers

- Snack: Roasted Chickpeas

- Dessert: Chocolate Avocado Pudding

Day 17

- Breakfast: Zucchini Bread Muffins

- Lunch: Grilled Chicken Breast with Steamed Broccoli

- Dinner: Lemon Herb Baked Cod with Steamed Broccoli

- Snack: Carrot Sticks with Avocado Dip

- Dessert: Peach Sorbet

Day 18

- Breakfast: Egg White Scramble with Spinach and Bell Peppers

- Lunch: Vegetable Stir-Fry with Tofu

- Dinner: Garlic Olive Oil Pasta with Spinach

- Snack: Apple Slices with Almond Butter

- Dessert: Rice Pudding

Day 19

- Breakfast: Low-Sodium Oatmeal with Apples and Cinnamon

- Lunch: Quinoa Salad with Chickpeas and Cucumbers

- Dinner: Baked Chicken with Roasted Carrots and Parsnips

- Snack: Baked Kale Chips

- Dessert: Vanilla and Almond Mousse

Day 20

- Breakfast: Cottage Cheese with Pineapple

- Lunch: Roasted Turkey and Avocado Wrap

- Dinner: Salmon Salad with Mixed Greens

- Snack: Zucchini Muffins

- Dessert: Carrot Cake Muffins

Day 21

- Breakfast: Blueberry Almond Breakfast Quinoa

- Lunch: Tuna Salad Sandwich on Whole Wheat Bread

- Dinner: Chicken and Broccoli Stir-Fry

- Snack: Rice Cakes with Cottage Cheese and Cherry Tomatoes

- Dessert: Angel Food Cake with Fresh Berries

Week 4

Day 22

- Breakfast: Almond Butter and Banana Sandwich

- Lunch: Cauliflower Rice Stir-Fry

- Dinner: Beef and Mushroom Skillet

- Snack: Greek Yogurt with Berries

- Dessert: Baked Pears with Honey and Walnuts

Day 23

- Breakfast: Spinach and Mushroom Omelette

- Lunch: Beet and Goat Cheese Arugula Salad

- Dinner: Shrimp and Asparagus Risotto

- Snack: Peanut Butter Banana Roll-Ups

- Dessert: Strawberry Banana Smoothie

Day 24

- Breakfast: Apple Cinnamon Baked Oatmeal

- Lunch: Turkey and Avocado Wrap

- Dinner: Vegetable Lentil Stew

- Snack: Avocado Toast with Egg

- Dessert: Lemon Ricotta Blueberry Cupcakes

Day 25

- Breakfast: Repeat your favorite breakfast

- Lunch: Grilled Veggie and Hummus Sandwich

- Dinner: Baked Lemon Pepper Tilapia

- Snack: Cucumber and Hummus Bites

- Dessert: Almond Joy Bars (Kidney-Friendly Version)

Day 26

- Breakfast: Cottage Cheese with Pineapple

- Lunch: Spinach and Goat Cheese Salad

- Dinner: Garlic Olive Oil Pasta with Spinach

- Snack: Boiled Eggs

- Dessert: Chocolate Avocado Pudding

Day 27

- Breakfast: Banana Yogurt Smoothie

- Lunch: Lentil Soup

- Dinner: Grilled Vegetable Platter

- Snack: Greek Yogurt with Berries

- Dessert: Peach Sorbet

Day 28

- Breakfast: Zucchini Bread Muffins

- Lunch: Quinoa Salad with Chickpeas and Cucumbers

- Dinner: Lemon Herb Baked Cod with Steamed Broccoli

- Snack: Carrot Sticks with Avocado Dip

- Dessert: Vanilla and Almond Mousse

Chapter 6

Breakfast Recipes for Kidney Health

Low-Sodium Oatmeal with Apples and Cinnamon

Ingredients:

- 1 cup rolled oats
- 2 cups water
- 1 apple, peeled and diced
- 1 tsp cinnamon
- 1 tbsp honey (optional)

Instructions:

1. Bring water to a boil in a saucepan. Add oats and reduce heat.
2. Simmer for 5 minutes, stirring occasionally.
3. Add diced apple and cinnamon. Cook for another 5 minutes.
4. Sweeten with honey if desired.

Nutritional Information:

- Low in sodium and potassium.
- High in fiber.

Egg White Scramble with Spinach and Bell Peppers

Ingredients:

- 4 egg whites
- 1 cup fresh spinach
- 1/2 bell pepper, diced
- Olive oil spray

Instructions:

1. Spray a non-stick pan with olive oil and heat.
2. Add bell pepper and sauté until soft.
3. Add spinach and cook until wilted.
4. Add egg whites and scramble until cooked.

Nutritional Information:

- Low in potassium and phosphorus.
- High in protein.

Blueberry Almond Breakfast Quinoa

Ingredients:

- 1 cup quinoa, rinsed
- 2 cups water
- 1/2 cup fresh blueberries
- 1/4 cup sliced almonds
- 1 tbsp maple syrup (optional)

Instructions:

1. In a saucepan, bring quinoa and water to a boil. Reduce heat and simmer, covered, for 15 minutes.
2. Remove from heat and let stand for 5 minutes. Fluff with a fork.
3. Top with blueberries, and almonds, and drizzle with maple syrup if desired.

Nutritional Information:

- Low in sodium and phosphorus.
- Provides healthy fats and protein.

Avocado Toast on Whole Grain Bread

Ingredients:

- 1 ripe avocado
- 2 slices whole grain bread, toasted
- Lemon juice
- Black pepper

Instructions:

1. Mash the avocado in a bowl. Add lemon juice and black pepper to taste.
2. Spread the avocado mixture on toasted bread slices.

Nutritional Information:

- High in healthy fats and fiber.
- Low in sodium and potassium.

Banana Yogurt Smoothie

Ingredients:

- 1 banana

- 1 cup low-fat Greek yogurt
- 1/2 cup ice
- 1/2 cup water or almond milk

Instructions:

1. Blend all ingredients until smooth.

Nutritional Information:

- High in protein and calcium.
- Low in phosphorus and sodium.

Cottage Cheese with Pineapple

Ingredients:

- 1/2 cup low-sodium cottage cheese
- 1/2 cup diced pineapple (fresh or canned in juice)

Instructions:

1. Mix cottage cheese with diced pineapple.

Nutritional Information:

- High in protein.
- Low in sodium and potassium.

Zucchini Bread Muffins

Ingredients:

- 1 1/2 cups all-purpose flour
- 1/2 cup sugar
- 1 tsp baking soda
- 1 tsp cinnamon
- 2 eggs
- 1/2 cup unsweetened applesauce
- 1 cup grated zucchini

Instructions:

1. Mix dry ingredients. In a separate bowl, beat eggs and add applesauce and zucchini.
2. Combine wet and dry ingredients until just mixed.
3. Pour into muffin tins and bake at 350°F for 20-25 minutes.

Nutritional Information:

- Low in sodium and potassium.

71

- Source of fiber.

Turkey and Avocado Wrap

Ingredients:

- 1 whole grain wrap
- 2 slices low-sodium turkey breast
- 1/4 avocado, sliced
- Lettuce

Instructions:

1. Lay the wrap flat and layer turkey, avocado slices, and lettuce.
2. Roll the wrap tightly and cut it in half.

Nutritional Information:

- High in protein and healthy fats.
- Low in sodium and potassium.

Peach and Cottage Cheese Pancakes

Ingredients:

- 1 cup all-purpose flour
- 1 tsp baking powder

- 1/2 cup low-sodium cottage cheese
- 3/4 cup water
- 1 egg
- 1/2 cup diced peaches

Instructions:

1. Mix flour and baking powder. In another bowl, mix cottage cheese, water, and egg.
2. Combine wet and dry ingredients, then fold in peaches.
3. Cook on a hot griddle until bubbles form, then flip.

Nutritional Information:

- High in protein.
- Low in sodium and potassium.

Almond Butter and Banana Sandwich

Ingredients:

- 2 slices whole grain bread
- 2 tbsp almond butter
- 1 banana, sliced

Instructions:

1. Spread almond butter on bread slices.
2. Arrange banana slices over one slice and top with the other.

Nutritional Information:

- High in healthy fats and fiber.
- Low in sodium.

Spinach and Mushroom Omelette

Ingredients:

- 2 eggs
- 1/2 cup sliced mushrooms
- 1 cup spinach
- Olive oil spray

Instructions:

1. Spray skillet with olive oil and heat.
2. Sauté mushrooms until brown, add spinach until wilted.
3. Beat eggs and pour over vegetables, cooking until set.

Nutritional Information:

- High in protein and vitamins.
- Low in sodium and potassium.

Apple Cinnamon Baked Oatmeal

Ingredients:

- 2 cups rolled oats
- 1 tsp cinnamon
- 1 apple, diced
- 2 cups almond milk
- 1/4 cup maple syrup

Instructions:

1. Mix all ingredients and pour into a baking dish.
2. Bake at 375°F for 25-30 minutes.

Nutritional Information:

- High in fiber.
- Low in sodium and potassium.

Chapter 7

Lunch Recipes for Kidney Health

Quinoa Salad with Chickpeas and Cucumbers

Ingredients:

- 1 cup quinoa, cooked
- 1/2 cup chickpeas, rinsed and drained
- 1 cucumber, diced
- 1/4 cup red onion, finely chopped
- 2 tbsp olive oil
- 1 tbsp lemon juice
- Salt and pepper to taste

Instructions:

1. In a large bowl, combine cooked quinoa, chickpeas, cucumber, and red onion.
2. Whisk together olive oil and lemon juice, season with salt and pepper.

3. Toss the salad with the dressing.

Nutritional Information:

- Low in sodium and potassium.
- High in protein and fiber.

Grilled Chicken Breast with Steamed Broccoli

Ingredients:

- 1 chicken breast, boneless and skinless
- 1 cup broccoli florets
- Olive oil
- Garlic powder
- Salt and pepper to taste

Instructions:

1. Season the chicken breast with garlic powder, salt, and pepper. Grill until cooked through.
2. Steam broccoli until tender.
3. Serve the chicken with steamed broccoli on the side.

Nutritional Information:

- High in protein.
- Low in sodium and potassium.

Vegetable Stir-Fry with Tofu

Ingredients:

- 1 cup tofu, cubed
- 2 cups mixed vegetables (carrots, bell peppers, and snap peas)
- 1 tbsp olive oil
- 1 tbsp low-sodium soy sauce
- 1 tsp ginger, minced
- 1 garlic clove, minced

Instructions:

1. Heat olive oil in a pan. Add ginger and garlic, sauté for a minute.
2. Add tofu cubes, and cook until slightly golden.
3. Add vegetables and stir-fry until tender-crisp.

4. Stir in low-sodium soy sauce and cook for another minute.

Nutritional Information:

- Low in sodium.
- High in protein and fiber.

Tuna Salad Sandwich on Whole Wheat Bread

Ingredients:

- 1 can low-sodium tuna, drained
- 2 tbsp mayonnaise
- 1/4 cup celery, chopped
- 1/4 cup red onion, chopped
- Lettuce leaves
- 2 slices whole wheat bread

Instructions:

1. In a bowl, mix tuna with mayonnaise, celery, and red onion.
2. Place lettuce leaves on one slice of bread, top with the tuna mixture, then cover with the other slice.

Nutritional Information:

- Low in phosphorus and potassium.
- Source of omega-3 fatty acids.

Roasted Turkey and Avocado Wrap

Ingredients:

- 1 whole wheat tortilla
- 2 slices low-sodium roasted turkey
- 1/4 avocado, sliced
- Lettuce
- Tomato slices

Instructions:

1. Lay the tortilla flat and arrange turkey, avocado slices, lettuce, and tomato on top.
2. Roll up the tortilla and slice it in half.

Nutritional Information:

- Low in sodium and potassium.

- High in healthy fats.

Lentil Soup

Ingredients:

- 1 cup lentils, rinsed
- 4 cups low-sodium vegetable broth
- 1 carrot, diced
- 1 celery stalk, diced
- 1 onion, chopped
- 2 garlic cloves, minced
- 1 tsp thyme
- Olive oil

Instructions:

1. In a pot, heat olive oil over medium heat. Add onion, garlic, carrot, and celery; cook until softened.
2. Add lentils, vegetable broth, and thyme. Bring to a boil, then simmer until lentils are tender.

Nutritional Information:

- Low in sodium and potassium.
- High in protein and fiber.

Grilled Veggie and Hummus Sandwich

Ingredients:

- 2 slices whole grain bread
- 1/4 cup hummus
- 1/4 cup grilled vegetables (zucchini, bell pepper, and eggplant)
- Spinach leaves

Instructions:

1. Spread hummus on both slices of bread.
2. Layer grilled vegetables and spinach leaves between the bread slices.

Nutritional Information:

- High in fiber.

- Low in sodium and potassium.

Spinach and Goat Cheese Salad

Ingredients:
- 2 cups fresh spinach
- 1/4 cup crumbled goat cheese
- 1/4 cup walnuts, chopped
- 1/4 cup dried cranberries
- 2 tbsp balsamic vinaigrette

Instructions:
1. In a large bowl, combine spinach, goat cheese, walnuts, and cranberries.
2. Drizzle with balsamic vinaigrette and toss gently.

Nutritional Information:
- Low in potassium and phosphorus.
- High in antioxidants.

Baked Salmon with Asparagus

Ingredients:

- 1 salmon fillet
- 1 cup asparagus spears
- Olive oil
- Lemon slices
- Salt and pepper to taste

Instructions:

1. Place salmon and asparagus on a baking sheet. Drizzle with olive oil and season with salt and pepper.
2. Top salmon with lemon slices.
3. Bake at 375°F for 20-25 minutes.

Nutritional Information:

- High in omega-3 fatty acids.
- Low in sodium and phosphorus.

Cauliflower Rice Stir-Fry

Ingredients:

- 2 cups cauliflower rice
- 1 cup mixed vegetables (peas, carrots, and bell peppers)
- 1 tbsp olive oil
- 1 egg, beaten
- 1 tbsp low-sodium soy sauce
- Green onions for garnish

Instructions:

1. Heat olive oil in a pan. Add mixed vegetables and stir-fry until soft.
2. Add cauliflower rice, and cook for 5 minutes.
3. Push the mixture to one side, pour the beaten egg on the other side, and scramble.
4. Mix everything, add soy sauce, and garnish with green onions.

Nutritional Information:

- Low in sodium and potassium.
- High in vitamins and fiber.

Beet and Goat Cheese Arugula Salad

Ingredients:

- 2 cups arugula
- 1/2 cup roasted beets, sliced
- 1/4 cup crumbled goat cheese
- 1/4 cup walnuts, toasted
- 2 tbsp olive oil
- 1 tbsp lemon juice

Instructions:

1. Combine arugula, beets, goat cheese, and walnuts in a bowl.
2. Whisk together olive oil and lemon juice, and drizzle over the salad.

Nutritional Information:

- Low in sodium and potassium.
- High in antioxidants and healthy fats.

Chicken and Avocado Salad

Ingredients:

- 1 cup cooked chicken breast, shredded
- 1 avocado, diced
- 1/2 cup cherry tomatoes, halved
- 1/4 cup cucumber, diced
- 1/4 cup red onion, finely chopped
- 2 tbsp cilantro, chopped
- 2 tbsp lime juice
- Salt and pepper to taste

Instructions:

1. In a large bowl, combine chicken, avocado, tomatoes, cucumber, red onion, and cilantro.
2. Drizzle with lime juice, season with salt and pepper, and toss well.

Nutritional Information:

- Low in sodium and potassium.
- High in healthy fats and protein.

Chapter 8

Dinner Recipes for Kidney Health

Lemon Herb Baked Cod

Ingredients:

- 4 cod fillets
- 2 tbsp olive oil
- 1 tbsp lemon juice
- 1 tsp dried herbs (thyme, oregano)
- Lemon slices for garnish
- Salt and pepper to taste

Instructions:

1. Preheat oven to 400°F (200°C).
2. Mix olive oil, lemon juice, herbs, salt, and pepper. Brush over cod fillets.
3. Place fillets in a baking dish, and top with lemon slices.
4. Bake for 12-15 minutes, until fish flakes easily.

Nutritional Information:

- Low in potassium and phosphorus.
- High in protein.

Grilled Vegetable Platter

Ingredients:

- 1 zucchini, sliced
- 1 bell pepper, cut into strips
- 1 eggplant, sliced
- 2 tbsp olive oil
- 1 tbsp balsamic vinegar
- Salt and pepper to taste

Instructions:

1. Preheat grill to medium-high.
2. Toss vegetables with olive oil, balsamic vinegar, salt, and pepper.
3. Grill vegetables until tender and slightly charred, turning occasionally.

Nutritional Information:

- Low in sodium, potassium, and phosphorus.
- High in fiber and antioxidants.

Garlic Olive Oil Pasta with Spinach

Ingredients:

- 8 oz whole wheat spaghetti
- 2 tbsp olive oil
- 2 garlic cloves, minced
- 2 cups fresh spinach
- Salt and pepper to taste
- Grated Parmesan cheese (optional)

Instructions:

1. Cook pasta according to package instructions; drain.
2. In a large pan, heat olive oil over medium heat. Add garlic and sauté until fragrant.

3. Add spinach and sauté until wilted. Toss with cooked pasta.

4. Season with salt and pepper. Serve with grated Parmesan if desired.

Nutritional Information:

- Low in sodium and potassium.
- High in fiber.

Turkey and Quinoa Stuffed Peppers

Ingredients:

- 4 bell peppers, halved and seeds removed
- 1 lb ground turkey
- 1 cup cooked quinoa
- 1 cup low-sodium tomato sauce
- 1 onion, chopped
- 1 tsp garlic powder
- 1 tsp cumin
- Olive oil

Instructions:

1. Preheat oven to 375°F (190°C).
2. In a skillet, heat olive oil over medium heat. Add onion and ground turkey, and cook until browned.
3. Stir in cooked quinoa, tomato sauce, garlic powder, and cumin.
4. Stuff bell peppers with the turkey mixture. Place in a baking dish.
5. Bake for 25-30 minutes, until peppers are tender.

Nutritional Information:

- Low in sodium and phosphorus.
- High in protein and fiber.

Baked Chicken with Roasted Carrots and Parsnips

Ingredients:

- 4 chicken thighs, skinless
- 4 carrots, sliced
- 4 parsnips, sliced

- 2 tbsp olive oil
- 1 tsp rosemary
- Salt and pepper to taste

Instructions:

1. Preheat oven to 425°F (220°C).
2. Toss carrots and parsnips with 1 tbsp olive oil, rosemary, salt, and pepper. Spread on a baking sheet.
3. Rub chicken with remaining olive oil, and season with salt and pepper. Place among the vegetables.
4. Bake for 35-40 minutes, until chicken is cooked through and vegetables are tender.

Nutritional Information:

- Low in potassium.
- High in protein and fiber.

Salmon Salad with Mixed Greens

Ingredients:

- 2 salmon fillets
- 4 cups mixed greens
- 1/2 cucumber, sliced
- 1/4 red onion, thinly sliced
- 2 tbsp olive oil
- 1 tbsp lemon juice
- Salt and pepper to taste

Instructions:

1. Grill salmon until cooked through and flaky.
2. Toss mixed greens, cucumber, and red onion with olive oil, lemon juice, salt, and pepper.
3. Top salad with grilled salmon.

Nutritional Information:

- Low in sodium and phosphorus.
- High in omega-3 fatty acids and protein.

Chicken and Broccoli Stir-Fry

Ingredients:

- 1 lb chicken breast, thinly sliced
- 2 cups broccoli florets
- 1 bell pepper, sliced
- 2 tbsp olive oil
- 2 tbsp low-sodium soy sauce
- 1 tsp ginger, minced
- 1 garlic clove, minced

Instructions:

1. Heat olive oil in a large skillet over medium-high heat.
2. Add chicken, and cook until no longer pink. Remove from skillet.
3. Add broccoli and bell pepper to the skillet, and stir-fry until tender-crisp.
4. Return chicken to the skillet, and add soy sauce, ginger, and garlic. Stir to combine and heat through.

Nutritional Information:

- Low in sodium and potassium.
- High in protein and vitamins.

Beef and Mushroom Skillet

Ingredients:

- 1 lb lean beef, cut into strips
- 2 cups sliced mushrooms
- 1 onion, sliced
- 1 tbsp olive oil
- 1 tbsp Worcestershire sauce
- Salt and pepper to taste

Instructions:

1. Heat olive oil in a skillet over medium-high heat. Add beef strips, and cook until browned. Remove and set aside.
2. In the same skillet, add onion and mushrooms. Cook until tender.

3. Return beef to the skillet, add Worcestershire sauce, salt, and pepper. Cook until heated through.

Nutritional Information:

- Low in phosphorus and potassium.
- High in protein.

Vegetable Lentil Stew

Ingredients:

- 1 cup lentils, rinsed
- 4 cups low-sodium vegetable broth
- 2 carrots, diced
- 2 celery stalks, diced
- 1 onion, diced
- 2 tomatoes, diced
- 1 tsp thyme
- 1 tsp rosemary
- Salt and pepper to taste

Instructions:

1. In a large pot, combine lentils, vegetable broth, carrots, celery, onion, and tomatoes.
2. Bring to a boil, reduce heat to low, and simmer for 30-40 minutes, until lentils are tender.
3. Add thyme, rosemary, salt, and pepper. Cook for an additional 5 minutes.

Nutritional Information:

- Low in sodium and potassium.
- High in fiber and protein.

Eggplant Parmesan (Light Version)

Ingredients:

- 1 eggplant, sliced
- 2 cups low-sodium marinara sauce
- 1 cup shredded mozzarella cheese
- 1/4 cup grated Parmesan cheese

- Olive oil spray
- Salt and pepper to taste

Instructions:

1. Preheat oven to 375°F (190°C). Spray eggplant slices with olive oil, and season with salt and pepper.
2. Bake eggplant slices until tender, about 20 minutes.
3. In a baking dish, layer marinara sauce, baked eggplant, mozzarella, and Parmesan cheese. Repeat layers.
4. Bake for 25-30 minutes, until cheese is bubbly and golden.

Nutritional Information:

- Low in sodium and potassium.
- Source of calcium and fiber.

Shrimp and Asparagus Risotto

Ingredients:

- 1 cup arborio rice
- 4 cups low-sodium chicken broth
- 1 lb shrimp, peeled and deveined
- 2 cups asparagus, chopped
- 1/2 onion, chopped
- 2 tbsp olive oil
- 1/4 cup grated Parmesan cheese
- Salt and pepper to taste

Instructions:

1. In a large pan, heat olive oil over medium heat. Add onion, and cook until translucent.
2. Add arborio rice, and cook for 1-2 minutes. Add chicken broth, 1 cup at a time, stirring frequently, until absorbed.

3. Add asparagus in the last 5 minutes of cooking. Add shrimp, and cook until they turn pink.
4. Stir in Parmesan cheese, and season with salt and pepper.

Nutritional Information:

- Low in sodium and potassium.
- High in protein.

Baked Lemon Pepper Tilapia

Ingredients:

- 4 tilapia fillets
- 2 tbsp olive oil
- 1 tbsp lemon pepper seasoning
- Lemon slices for garnish

Instructions:

1. Preheat oven to 400°F (200°C).
2. Place tilapia on a baking sheet, drizzle with olive oil, and sprinkle with lemon pepper seasoning.

3. Bake for 10-12 minutes, until fish flakes easily.

4. Garnish with lemon slices.

Nutritional Information:

- Low in sodium and potassium.
- High in protein.

Chapter 9

Snacks Recipes for Kidney Health

Cucumber and Hummus Bites

Ingredients:

- 1 large cucumber, sliced
- 1 cup hummus

Instructions:

1. Slice cucumber into thick rounds.
2. Top each cucumber round with a spoonful of hummus.

Nutritional Information:

- Low in sodium and potassium.
- High in fiber.

Apple Slices with Almond Butter

Ingredients:

- 1 apple, cored and sliced
- 2 tbsp almond butter

Instructions:

1. Core and slice the apple.
2. Spread almond butter on each apple slice.

Nutritional Information:

- Low in sodium.
- Provides healthy fats and fiber.

Carrot Sticks with Avocado Dip

Ingredients:

- 2 carrots, peeled and cut into sticks
- 1 ripe avocado
- 1 tbsp lime juice
- Salt and pepper to taste

Instructions:

1. Mash the avocado in a bowl and mix with lime juice, salt, and pepper.
2. Serve carrot sticks with the avocado dip.

Nutritional Information:

- Low in sodium and potassium.
- High in healthy fats and fiber.

Baked Kale Chips

Ingredients:

- 1 bunch kale, washed and torn into pieces
- 1 tbsp olive oil
- Salt to taste

Instructions:

1. Preheat oven to 350°F (175°C).
2. Toss kale pieces with olive oil and salt.
3. Spread on a baking sheet and bake for 10-15 minutes until crispy.

Nutritional Information:

- Low in sodium and potassium.
- High in vitamins A and C.

Zucchini Muffins

Ingredients:

- 1 1/2 cups whole wheat flour
- 1 tsp baking powder
- 1/2 tsp baking soda
- 1 tsp cinnamon
- 2 eggs
- 1/4 cup olive oil
- 1/2 cup unsweetened applesauce
- 1 cup grated zucchini
- 1/4 cup honey

Instructions:

1. Preheat oven to 350°F (175°C).
2. Mix dry ingredients. In another bowl, beat eggs, olive oil, applesauce, and honey.
3. Combine wet and dry ingredients, and fold in zucchini.
4. Pour batter into muffin tins and bake for 20 minutes.

Nutritional Information:

- Low in sodium.
- Source of fiber and vitamins.

Rice Cakes with Cottage Cheese and Cherry Tomatoes

Ingredients:

- Rice cakes
- Low-sodium cottage cheese
- Cherry tomatoes, sliced

Instructions:

1. Spread cottage cheese on rice cakes.
2. Top with sliced cherry tomatoes.

Nutritional Information:

- Low in sodium and potassium.
- High in protein.

Roasted Chickpeas

Ingredients:

- 1 can chickpeas, rinsed and drained

- 1 tbsp olive oil
- 1/2 tsp garlic powder
- Salt to taste

Instructions:

1. Preheat oven to 400°F (200°C).
2. Toss chickpeas with olive oil, garlic powder, and salt.
3. Spread on a baking sheet and roast for 20-30 minutes until crispy.

Nutritional Information:

- Low in potassium.
- High in protein and fiber.

Greek Yogurt with Berries

Ingredients:

- 1 cup low-fat Greek yogurt
- 1/2 cup mixed berries (strawberries, blueberries)

Instructions:

1. Top Greek yogurt with mixed berries.

Nutritional Information:

- Low in sodium.
- High in protein and calcium.

Boiled Eggs

Ingredients:

- Eggs

Instructions:

1. Boil eggs to your liking (soft-boiled or hard-boiled).
2. Peel and serve.

Nutritional Information:

- Low in sodium and potassium.
- High in protein.

Peanut Butter Banana Roll-Ups

Ingredients:

- Whole wheat tortillas
- 2 tbsp peanut butter
- 1 banana, sliced

Instructions:

1. Spread peanut butter on tortillas.
2. Place banana slices on top and roll up.

Nutritional Information:

- Provides healthy fats and fiber.
- Low in sodium.

Avocado Toast with Egg

Ingredients:

- 1 slice whole grain bread, toasted
- 1/2 avocado, mashed
- 1 egg, cooked to your preference

Instructions:

1. Spread mashed avocado on toasted bread.
2. Top with cooked egg.

Nutritional Information:

- High in healthy fats and protein.
- Low in sodium.

Veggie Sticks with Greek Yogurt Ranch Dip

Ingredients for Dip:

- 1 cup low-fat Greek yogurt
- 1 tsp dried dill
- 1 tsp garlic powder
- 1 tsp onion powder
- Salt and pepper to taste

Ingredients for Veggie Sticks:

- Carrots, celery, bell peppers, cut into sticks

Instructions:

1. Mix Greek yogurt with dill, garlic powder, onion powder, salt, and pepper.
2. Serve dip with veggie sticks.

Nutritional Information:

- Dip is low in sodium and potassium.
- High in protein.

Chapter 10

Dessert Recipes for Kidney Health

Berry and Yogurt Parfait

Ingredients:

- 1 cup low-fat Greek yogurt

- 1/2 cup mixed berries (strawberries, blueberries)

- 2 tbsp granola (low sodium)

Instructions:

1. Layer half of the yogurt in a glass.

2. Add a layer of mixed berries, then a layer of granola.

3. Repeat the layers with the remaining ingredients.

Nutritional Information:

- Low in sodium and phosphorus.

- High in calcium and antioxidants.

Apple Cinnamon Baked Apples

Ingredients:

- 4 apples, cored

- 2 tbsp brown sugar

- 1 tsp cinnamon

- 1/4 cup raisins

- 1/4 cup water

Instructions:

1. Preheat oven to 350°F (175°C).

2. Mix brown sugar, cinnamon, and raisins. Stuff each apple with the mixture.

3. Place apples in a baking dish, and add water to the bottom.

4. Bake for 30-35 minutes, until apples are soft.

Nutritional Information:

- Low in sodium.

- Source of fiber.

Angel Food Cake with Fresh Berries

Ingredients:

- 1 store-bought angel food cake

- 1 cup mixed berries (strawberries, blueberries, raspberries)

- 2 tbsp honey

Instructions:

1. Slice the angel food cake.

2. Top each slice with mixed berries.

3. Drizzle honey over the berries and cake.

Nutritional Information:

- Low in phosphorus and sodium.

- Low in fat.

Peach Sorbet

Ingredients:

- 4 cups frozen peaches

- 1/4 cup honey

- 1/2 cup water

Instructions:

1. Blend frozen peaches, honey, and water in a blender until smooth.

2. Freeze the mixture until set, about 2-3 hours.

Nutritional Information:

- No added sodium.

- Source of vitamins.

Rice Pudding

Ingredients:

- 1/2 cup uncooked white rice

- 2 cups low-fat milk

- 1/4 cup sugar

- 1 tsp vanilla extract

- Cinnamon to taste

Instructions:

1. In a saucepan, combine rice and milk. Bring to a boil, then reduce heat to low.

2. Simmer until rice is tender and milk is mostly absorbed, stirring occasionally.

3. Stir in sugar and vanilla extract. Serve with a sprinkle of cinnamon.

Nutritional Information:

- Low in sodium and phosphorus.

- Source of calcium.

Vanilla and Almond Mousse

Ingredients:

- 1 cup low-fat Greek yogurt

- 1 tsp vanilla extract

- 2 tbsp almond butter

- 1 tbsp honey

Instructions:

1. Mix Greek yogurt, vanilla extract, almond butter, and honey until smooth.

2. Chill in the refrigerator for at least 1
    hour before serving.

Nutritional Information:

- Low in sodium.

- High in protein and healthy fats.

Carrot Cake Muffins

Ingredients:

- 1 1/2 cups whole wheat flour

- 1 tsp baking powder

- 1/2 tsp baking soda

- 1 tsp cinnamon

- 1/4 cup olive oil

- 1/2 cup honey

- 2 eggs

- 1 cup grated carrots

Instructions:

1. Preheat oven to 350°F (175°C).

2. Mix dry ingredients. In another bowl, beat eggs, olive oil, and honey.

3. Combine wet and dry ingredients, and fold in carrots.

4. Pour batter into muffin tins and bake for 20 minutes.

Nutritional Information:

- Low in sodium.

- Source of fiber.

Chocolate Avocado Pudding

Ingredients:

- 2 ripe avocados

- 1/4 cup cocoa powder

- 1/4 cup honey

- 1/2 cup milk (or almond milk)

- 1 tsp vanilla extract

Instructions:

1. Blend avocados, cocoa powder, honey, milk, and vanilla extract until smooth.

2. Chill in the refrigerator for at least 1 hour before serving.

Nutritional Information:

- Low in sodium and potassium.

- High in healthy fats.

Baked Pears with Honey and Walnuts

Ingredients:

- 4 pears, halved and cored

- 2 tbsp honey

- 1/2 cup chopped walnuts

- Cinnamon to taste

Instructions:

1. Preheat oven to 350°F (175°C).

2. Place pear halves on a baking sheet. Drizzle with honey, and sprinkle with walnuts and cinnamon.

3. Bake for 25-30 minutes, until pears are soft.

Nutritional Information:

- Low in sodium.

- Source of omega-3 fatty acids and fiber.

Strawberry Banana Smoothie

Ingredients:

- 1 banana

- 1 cup strawberries

- 1 cup low-fat Greek yogurt

- 1/2 cup water or almond milk

Instructions:

1. Blend banana, strawberries, Greek yogurt, and water (or almond milk) until smooth.

Nutritional Information:

- Low in sodium and phosphorus.

- High in protein and vitamin C.

Lemon Ricotta Blueberry Cupcakes

Ingredients:

- 1 1/2 cups all-purpose flour

- 1 tsp baking powder

- 1/2 cup low-fat ricotta cheese

- 3/4 cup sugar

- 2 eggs

- 1/2 tsp vanilla extract

- 1 tbsp lemon zest

- 1 cup blueberries

Instructions:

1. Preheat oven to 350°F (175°C).

2. Mix dry ingredients. In another bowl, beat eggs, ricotta, sugar, vanilla, and lemon zest.

3. Combine wet and dry ingredients, and fold in blueberries.

4. Pour batter into cupcake tins and bake for 20-25 minutes.

Nutritional Information:

- Low in sodium.

- Source of antioxidants.

124

Almond Joy Bars (Kidney-Friendly Version)

Ingredients:

- 1 cup shredded unsweetened coconut

- 1/3 cup almond butter

- 1/4 cup honey

- 1/4 cup chopped almonds

- 1/2 cup melted dark chocolate (at least 70% cocoa)

Instructions:

1. Mix coconut, almond butter, and honey until well combined. Press into the bottom of a lined pan.

2. Sprinkle chopped almonds over the coconut layer. Pour melted chocolate over the top.

125

3. Chill in the refrigerator until set, then cut into bars.

Nutritional Information:

- Low in sodium and phosphorus.

- High in healthy fats and antioxidants.

Chapter 11

Conclusion

Creating a comprehensive food list and guide for individuals with kidney disease is an invaluable tool for managing health, promoting kidney function, and enhancing overall well-being. This guide serves not only as a dietary framework but also as a pathway to a healthier lifestyle for those facing kidney health challenges. Focusing on kidney-friendly foods—those low in sodium, potassium, phosphorus, and protein, where necessary provides a blueprint for nutritional intake that supports kidney health and can help manage the progression of kidney disease.

The inclusion of specific food categories such as fruits, vegetables, grains, protein sources, and dairy alternatives, along with tailored recipes for breakfast, lunch, dinner, snacks, and desserts, caters to a variety of tastes and dietary needs, ensuring that individuals can enjoy delicious and nutritious meals without compromising their health. The guide emphasizes the importance of balance, moderation, and the need for personalized dietary planning, considering that every individual's condition and nutritional requirements can vary significantly based on the stage of kidney disease and other health factors.

A key takeaway from this food guide is the critical role that diet plays in managing kidney disease and improving quality of life. By making informed choices about the foods consumed, individuals can take proactive steps toward maintaining their kidney health and preventing further complications. Those with kidney disease need to consult with healthcare professionals, including dietitians specialized in renal nutrition, to create a diet plan that's tailored to their specific needs, ensuring that they receive the right balance of nutrients without overburdening their kidneys.

Ultimately, this guide serves as a testament to the power of dietary management in the context of kidney disease. It stands as a resource for patients, caregivers, and healthcare providers alike, offering guidance, inspiration, and practical solutions for eating well with kidney disease. With the right approach to nutrition, individuals with kidney disease can lead fulfilling lives, demonstrating that with careful planning and consideration, dietary restrictions can transform into a varied and enjoyable eating plan that supports kidney health and overall wellness.

BONUS

Lifestyle Changes for Better Kidney Health

Improving kidney health involves more than just dietary adjustments. A holistic approach that includes various lifestyle changes can significantly enhance kidney function and overall well-being.

Here are key lifestyle changes that can contribute to better kidney health:

1. Maintain a Healthy Weight

Achieving and maintaining a healthy weight can reduce the risk of developing conditions like diabetes and hypertension, which can lead to kidney damage. Consider regular physical activity and a balanced diet as part of your weight management strategy.

2. Stay Active

Regular physical activity helps control blood pressure, reduce stress, and maintain a healthy weight. Activities like walking, swimming, cycling, and yoga can be beneficial. Always consult with your healthcare provider before starting any new exercise program, especially if you have existing health conditions.

3. Monitor Blood Pressure

High blood pressure is a leading cause of kidney damage. Manage your blood pressure through a healthy diet, regular exercise, limiting alcohol intake, avoiding tobacco, and stress management. If you have high blood pressure, adhere to your prescribed medication regimen.

4. Control Blood Sugar Levels

Diabetes is another major risk factor for kidney disease. If you have diabetes, managing your blood sugar levels through diet, exercise, and medication (if prescribed) is crucial to prevent kidney damage.

5. Stay Hydrated

Adequate hydration helps your kidneys clear sodium, urea, and toxins from the body. Drinking enough water is generally beneficial, but it's essential to adjust your fluid intake if your kidney function is impaired or if you have been advised to limit fluids by your healthcare provider.

6. Quit Smoking

Smoking damages blood vessels, which can decrease the flow of blood to the kidneys. Quitting smoking can improve your kidney health and reduce your risk of kidney disease.

7. Limit Alcohol Consumption

Excessive alcohol consumption can cause changes in the kidneys and increase blood pressure. Limiting alcohol to moderate levels is advised to protect your kidneys.

8. Avoid Overuse of Over-the-Counter Painkillers

Regular use of non-steroidal anti-inflammatory drugs (NSAIDs) like ibuprofen and naproxen can cause kidney damage. Use these medications minimally and only as directed.

9. Get Regular Kidney Function Checks

Regular screenings can help detect kidney function decline early, especially if you're at risk due to diabetes, hypertension, or a family history of kidney disease. Early detection can lead to more effective management.

10. Manage Stress

Chronic stress can lead to high blood pressure and other behaviors that increase the risk of kidney damage, such as poor dietary choices and excessive alcohol consumption. Find stress-reduction techniques that work for you, such as meditation, deep breathing exercises, and engaging in hobbies.

11. Sleep Well

Adequate sleep is vital for overall health and helps regulate kidney function. Aim for 7-9 hours of quality sleep per night and maintain a regular sleep schedule.

12. Stay Informed and Supportive Network

Educate yourself about kidney health and stay updated on your condition. A supportive network of family, friends, and healthcare professionals can provide guidance, encouragement, and care.

Made in the USA
Columbia, SC
30 October 2024

e0382446-4e14-4b33-979f-1aefe58af6d0R01